This publication is intended to provide educational information for the reader on the covered subjects. It is not intended to take the place of personalized medical counseling, diagnosis, and treatment from a trained healthcare professional.

ISBN 978-1-998740-21-5 (Paperback)

Printed and bound in USA
Published by Loons Press

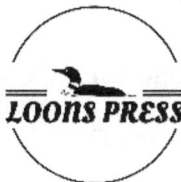

LOONS PRESS

Table Of Contents

How To Heal PCOS Naturally

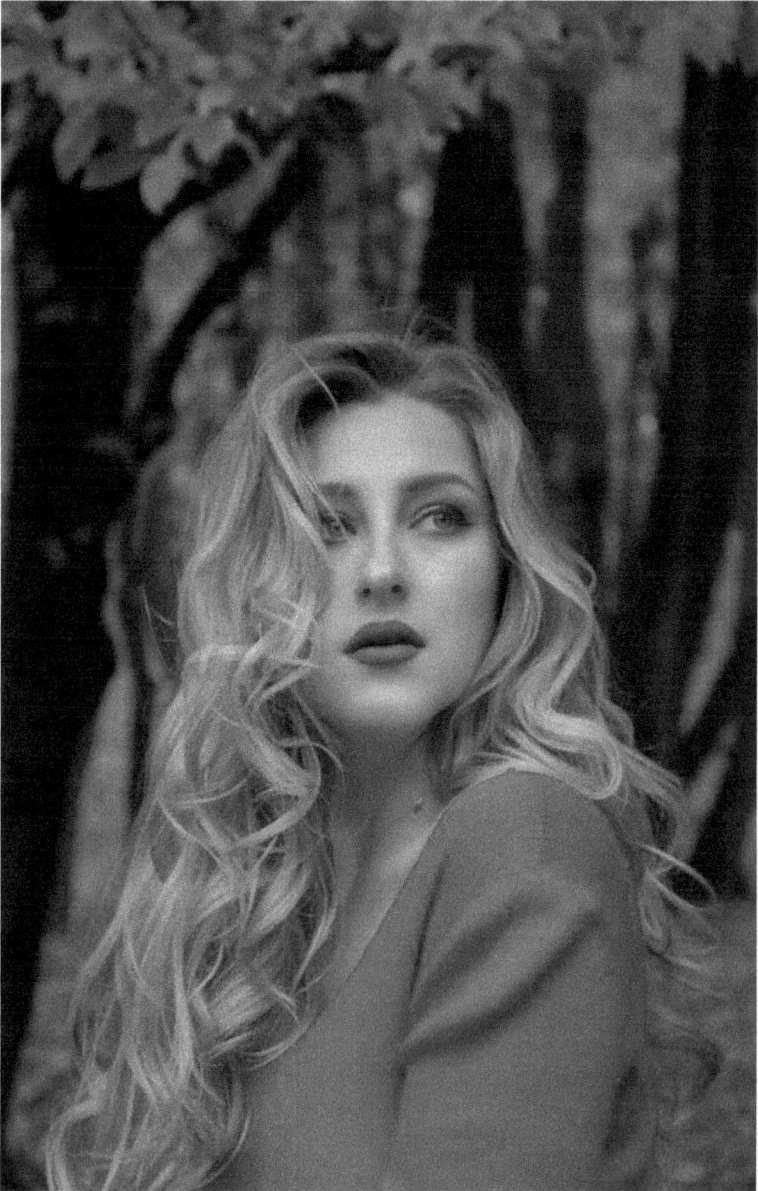

A Comprehensive Guide for Women

Chapter 1

Understanding PCOS

What is PCOS?

PCOS, or Polycystic Ovarian Syndrome, is a common hormonal disorder that affects women of reproductive age. It is estimated that up to 10% of women worldwide may have PCOS, making it one of the most common endocrine disorders in women. PCOS is characterized by a variety of symptoms, including irregular periods, acne, weight gain, and infertility. It is important for women with PCOS to understand the underlying causes of their condition in order to effectively manage their symptoms and improve their overall health.

One of the key factors in the development of PCOS is insulin resistance, which can lead to high levels of insulin in the blood. Insulin resistance can disrupt the balance of hormones in the body, leading to symptoms such as irregular periods and difficulty losing weight.

In addition, high levels of insulin can increase the production of androgens, or male hormones, which can contribute to symptoms such as acne and unwanted hair growth.

Another important factor in the development of PCOS is inflammation. Chronic inflammation in the body can worsen insulin resistance and disrupt hormone balance, leading to an increase in symptoms of PCOS. Inflammation can be caused by a variety of factors, including poor diet, stress, and environmental toxins. By reducing inflammation in the body, women with PCOS can help to improve their symptoms and overall health.

In addition to insulin resistance and inflammation, genetics may also play a role in the development of PCOS. Women with a family history of PCOS are more likely to develop the condition themselves. While genetics cannot be changed, lifestyle factors such as diet and exercise can help to manage symptoms and improve overall health in women with PCOS. By understanding the underlying causes of PCOS and making positive changes to their lifestyle, women with PCOS can take control of their health and work towards healing their condition naturally.

Overall, PCOS is a complex hormonal disorder that affects many women worldwide. By understanding the underlying causes of PCOS, such as insulin resistance, inflammation, and genetics, women with PCOS can take steps to manage their symptoms and improve their overall health.

Through lifestyle changes such as a healthy diet, regular exercise, and stress management, women with PCOS can work towards healing their condition naturally and improving their quality of life.

Causes of PCOS

PCOS, or Polycystic Ovarian Syndrome, is a common hormonal disorder that affects women of reproductive age. There are several factors that can contribute to the development of PCOS, including genetics, insulin resistance, and hormonal imbalances. Understanding the causes of PCOS is crucial in order to effectively manage and treat the condition.

One of the primary causes of PCOS is genetics. Women with a family history of PCOS are more likely to develop the condition themselves. This genetic predisposition can lead to hormonal imbalances and difficulties with insulin regulation, which are common symptoms of PCOS. While genetics play a significant role in the development of PCOS, lifestyle factors also play a crucial role in the management of the condition.

Insulin resistance is another common cause of PCOS. Insulin is a hormone that helps regulate blood sugar levels in the body. When the body becomes resistant to insulin, it can lead to an imbalance of hormones such as testosterone and estrogen, which can contribute to the development of PCOS. Managing insulin resistance through dietary changes, exercise, and stress reduction techniques can help improve symptoms of PCOS and promote overall health.

Hormonal imbalances are a hallmark of PCOS, with elevated levels of androgens (male hormones) such as testosterone being a common feature. These hormonal imbalances can disrupt the menstrual cycle, leading to irregular periods, infertility, and other symptoms associated with PCOS.

By addressing hormonal imbalances through lifestyle changes, such as improving diet and managing stress, women with PCOS can help regulate their hormones and improve their symptoms.

In addition to genetics, insulin resistance, and hormonal imbalances, other factors such as obesity, sedentary lifestyle, and poor diet can also contribute to the development of PCOS. By addressing these underlying causes through natural interventions such as dietary changes, exercise, and stress management techniques, women with PCOS can effectively manage their symptoms and improve their overall health. By understanding the causes of PCOS and taking a holistic approach to treatment, women can empower themselves to heal PCOS naturally and improve their quality of life.

Symptoms of PCOS

PCOS, or Polycystic Ovarian Syndrome, is a common hormonal disorder that affects women of reproductive age. One of the most important aspects of managing PCOS is understanding its symptoms.

By recognizing these symptoms early on, individuals can take proactive steps to manage their condition and improve their overall health.

One of the most common symptoms of PCOS is irregular menstrual cycles. Women with PCOS often experience infrequent or prolonged periods, which can make it difficult to predict ovulation and conceive. Additionally, many women with PCOS also experience heavy or painful periods, which can significantly impact their quality of life. If you have irregular menstrual cycles, it may be a sign that you have PCOS and should consult with a healthcare provider for further evaluation.

Another common symptom of PCOS is excessive hair growth, known as hirsutism. This excess hair growth is often found on the face, chest, back, or buttocks and can be embarrassing and distressing for many women. Hirsutism is caused by elevated levels of androgens, or male hormones, in the body, which is a hallmark of PCOS. By addressing the underlying hormonal imbalance, individuals with PCOS can reduce excessive hair growth and improve their self-esteem.

Weight gain and difficulty losing weight are also common symptoms of PCOS. Many women with PCOS struggle to maintain a healthy weight, despite following a balanced diet and regular exercise routine. This is because insulin resistance, a common feature of PCOS, can make it harder for the body to regulate blood sugar levels and store fat. By addressing insulin resistance through dietary changes and lifestyle modifications, individuals with PCOS can improve their metabolism and achieve a healthy weight.

In addition to these symptoms, many women with PCOS also experience acne, oily skin, and scalp hair loss. These skin and hair changes are often caused by elevated levels of androgens in the body, which can stimulate the production of sebum and clog pores. By addressing the underlying hormonal imbalance, individuals with PCOS can improve their skin and hair health and boost their self-confidence. Overall, recognizing and addressing the symptoms of PCOS is essential for managing the condition and improving overall health and well-being. By taking a holistic approach to healing PCOS naturally, individuals can address the root causes of their symptoms and achieve long-lasting relief.

Diagnosing PCOS

Diagnosing PCOS can be a complex and frustrating process for many women. The symptoms of Polycystic Ovarian Syndrome (PCOS) can vary widely from person to person, making it difficult to diagnose without a comprehensive evaluation. However, there are certain key indicators that healthcare providers look for when diagnosing PCOS.

One of the most common symptoms of PCOS is irregular periods or no periods at all. This is often due to hormonal imbalances that can disrupt the normal menstrual cycle. Other symptoms may include weight gain, acne, excessive hair growth (hirsutism), and hair loss. If you are experiencing any of these symptoms, it is important to speak with your healthcare provider to determine if PCOS may be the underlying cause.

In order to diagnose PCOS, your healthcare provider will likely perform a physical exam and take a detailed medical history. They may also order blood tests to check hormone levels, as well as an ultrasound to look for cysts on the ovaries.

It is important to be honest and thorough when discussing your symptoms with your healthcare provider, as this will help them make an accurate diagnosis.

It is important to note that there is no one-size-fits-all approach to diagnosing PCOS. Some women may have all of the classic symptoms, while others may only have a few. Additionally, PCOS can present differently in each individual, making it important for healthcare providers to take a personalized approach to diagnosis and treatment.

If you have been diagnosed with PCOS, it is important to work closely with your healthcare provider to develop a treatment plan that works for you. This may include lifestyle changes such as diet and exercise, as well as medications to help regulate hormone levels. By taking a proactive approach to managing your PCOS, you can improve your symptoms and overall quality of life.

How To Heal PCOS Naturally

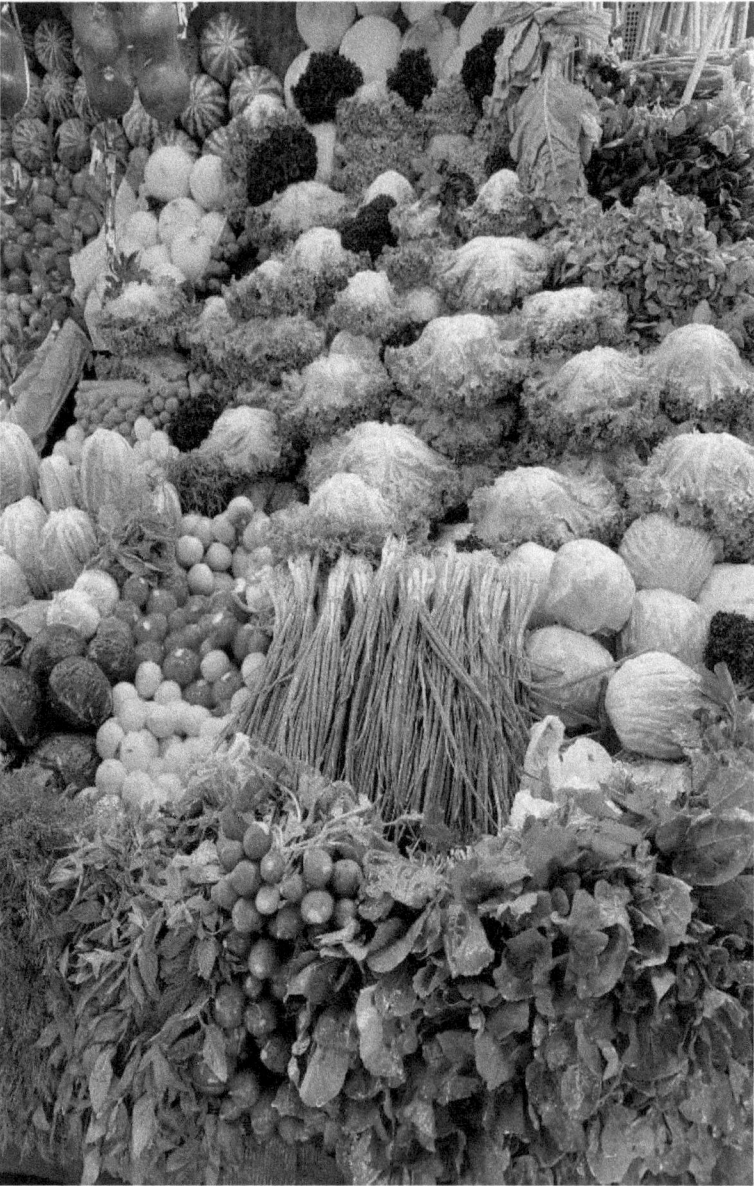

A Comprehensive Guide for Women

Chapter 2

Managing PCOS through Diet

Importance of Nutrition for PCOS

PCOS, or Polycystic Ovarian Syndrome, is a common hormonal disorder that affects many women worldwide. One of the key components in managing PCOS is nutrition. Eating a balanced diet that is rich in nutrients is crucial for women with PCOS to help manage their symptoms and improve their overall health.

By focusing on nutrition, women with PCOS can take control of their health and reduce the impact of this condition on their daily lives.

Nutrition plays a vital role in managing PCOS because it can help regulate insulin levels in the body. Many women with PCOS have insulin resistance, which can lead to weight gain and difficulty losing weight.

By following a diet that is low in refined carbohydrates and sugars, and high in fiber and protein, women with PCOS can help regulate their insulin levels and improve their overall health. This can lead to weight loss, improved energy levels, and a reduced risk of developing other health conditions associated with PCOS.

In addition to regulating insulin levels, nutrition is also important for managing other symptoms of PCOS, such as irregular periods and fertility issues. Eating a diet that is rich in vitamins, minerals, and antioxidants can help regulate hormone levels in the body and improve overall reproductive health. By focusing on nutrient-dense foods such as fruits, vegetables, whole grains, and lean proteins, women with PCOS can support their reproductive health and increase their chances of conceiving.

Furthermore, nutrition is essential for managing inflammation in the body, which is often elevated in women with PCOS. Inflammation can worsen symptoms of PCOS and lead to other health issues such as heart disease and diabetes.

By following an anti-inflammatory diet that is rich in omega-3 fatty acids, antioxidants, and phytonutrients, women with PCOS can reduce inflammation in their bodies and improve their overall health. This can lead to a reduction in symptoms, improved fertility, and a lower risk of developing other health conditions.

Overall, nutrition is a key component in managing PCOS naturally. By focusing on a balanced diet that is rich in nutrients and supports overall health, women with PCOS can take control of their symptoms and improve their quality of life.

Through proper nutrition, women with PCOS can reduce insulin resistance, regulate hormone levels, manage inflammation, and support their reproductive health. By making simple changes to their diet, women with PCOS can make a significant impact on their health and well-being.

Foods to Eat for PCOS

PCOS, or Polycystic Ovarian Syndrome, is a common hormonal disorder that affects many women. One of the key components of managing PCOS is through diet. By incorporating the right foods into your daily meals, you can help alleviate symptoms and promote overall wellness. In this subchapter, we will explore some of the best foods to eat for PCOS.

First and foremost, it is important to focus on whole, nutrient-dense foods. This includes plenty of fruits, vegetables, whole grains, and lean proteins. These foods are rich in vitamins, minerals, and antioxidants that can help regulate hormones and improve insulin sensitivity, which is crucial for managing PCOS symptoms.

One of the best foods to eat for PCOS is leafy greens such as spinach, kale, and collard greens. These vegetables are packed with nutrients like folate, magnesium, and fiber, which can help regulate insulin levels and reduce inflammation in the body.

Additionally, leafy greens are low in calories and high in water content, making them a great choice for weight management, which is often a concern for women with PCOS.

Another important food group for women with PCOS is healthy fats. Foods like avocados, nuts, seeds, and olive oil are rich in monounsaturated and polyunsaturated fats, which can help balance hormones and reduce inflammation in the body. These fats are also essential for proper hormone production and can help improve insulin sensitivity.

In addition to leafy greens and healthy fats, women with PCOS should incorporate plenty of lean proteins into their diet. Foods like chicken, fish, tofu, and legumes are all excellent sources of protein that can help stabilize blood sugar levels and promote satiety. Protein is also important for muscle growth and repair, which can help support overall health and wellness for women with PCOS.

Overall, a well-rounded diet that focuses on whole, nutrient-dense foods like leafy greens, healthy fats, and lean proteins is key for managing PCOS naturally. By making simple changes to your diet and incorporating these foods into your meals, you can help alleviate symptoms, regulate hormones, and promote overall wellness. Remember to consult with a healthcare provider or nutritionist before making any significant changes to your diet to ensure that it is appropriate for your individual needs and health goals.

Foods to Avoid for PCOS

PCOS, or Polycystic Ovarian Syndrome, is a hormonal disorder that affects many women worldwide. One of the key factors in managing PCOS is maintaining a healthy diet. There are certain foods that can exacerbate symptoms of PCOS and should be avoided in order to promote healing naturally.

One of the foods to avoid for PCOS is processed sugars. Foods high in refined sugars can cause spikes in blood sugar levels, leading to insulin resistance and weight gain - two common issues associated with PCOS.

By cutting back on sugary snacks and desserts, individuals with PCOS can better manage their symptoms and improve their overall health.

Another food to avoid for PCOS is refined carbohydrates. Foods such as white bread, pasta, and rice can also cause spikes in blood sugar levels and contribute to insulin resistance. Opting for whole grains like quinoa, brown rice, and whole wheat bread can help stabilize blood sugar levels and promote weight loss in individuals with PCOS.

Dairy products are also best avoided for individuals with PCOS. Dairy can be inflammatory for some people, leading to bloating, acne, and other symptoms. Switching to dairy alternatives like almond milk or coconut yogurt can help alleviate these symptoms and improve overall gut health, which is crucial for managing PCOS.

Additionally, individuals with PCOS should limit their intake of red meat and processed meats. These foods can be high in saturated fats, which can contribute to inflammation and weight gain.

Opting for lean proteins like chicken, fish, and plant-based proteins like tofu and legumes can help individuals with PCOS maintain a healthy weight and reduce inflammation in the body.

In conclusion, by avoiding processed sugars, refined carbohydrates, dairy products, and red and processed meats, individuals with PCOS can better manage their symptoms and promote healing naturally. Making small changes to diet and focusing on whole, nutrient-dense foods can have a significant impact on overall health and well-being for those with PCOS.

Sample PCOS-friendly Meal Plan

Eating a balanced and nutritious diet is essential for managing PCOS symptoms and promoting overall health. By making small changes to your eating habits, you can help regulate your hormones, improve insulin sensitivity, and reduce inflammation in the body. In this chapter, we will provide you with a sample PCOS-friendly meal plan to help you get started on your journey to healing PCOS naturally.

Breakfast:

Start your day with a healthy and filling breakfast to kickstart your metabolism and keep your energy levels stable throughout the morning. A good option for breakfast is a smoothie made with unsweetened almond milk, spinach, frozen berries, and a scoop of protein powder. You can also enjoy a bowl of Greek yogurt topped with nuts and seeds for added protein and healthy fats.

Lunch:

For lunch, aim to include a balance of protein, healthy fats, and complex carbohydrates to keep you satisfied and energized. A delicious lunch option is a grilled chicken salad with mixed greens, avocado, cherry tomatoes, and a drizzle of olive oil and balsamic vinegar. You can also try a quinoa and vegetable stir-fry with tofu for a plant-based protein option.

Snack:

It's important to have healthy snacks on hand to keep your blood sugar levels stable and prevent cravings for sugary or processed foods. A great snack option for PCOS is a handful of almonds and a piece of fruit, such as an apple or pear.

You can also enjoy a small serving of hummus with carrot sticks or cucumber slices for a satisfying and nutritious snack.

Dinner:

For dinner, focus on incorporating lean proteins, plenty of vegetables, and healthy fats into your meal. A tasty dinner option is grilled salmon with roasted sweet potatoes and steamed broccoli. You can also try a lentil and vegetable curry served with brown rice for a plant-based meal that is rich in fiber and nutrients.

Dessert:

If you have a sweet tooth, there are still plenty of PCOS-friendly dessert options to enjoy in moderation. A delicious dessert idea is a chia seed pudding made with unsweetened almond milk, chia seeds, and a touch of maple syrup or stevia for sweetness. You can also try a small serving of dark chocolate with a handful of raspberries for a decadent and satisfying treat.

By following this sample PCOS-friendly meal plan and making mindful choices about the foods you eat, you can support your body in healing naturally and managing your PCOS symptoms effectively. Remember to listen to your body's cues, eat mindfully, and make adjustments to your meal plan as needed to find what works best for you. With dedication and consistency, you can take control of your health and well-being and thrive with PCOS.

How To Heal PCOS Naturally

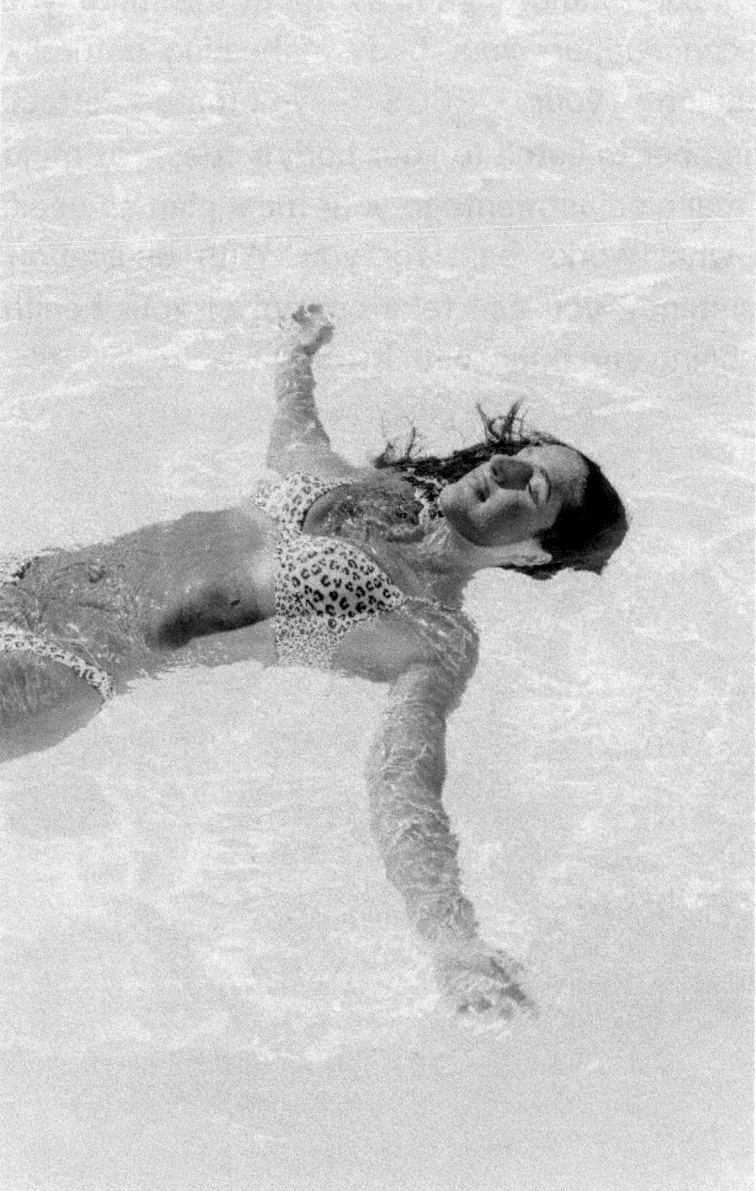

Chapter 3

Exercise and PCOS

Benefits of Exercise for PCOS

Exercise is a powerful tool for managing Polycystic Ovarian Syndrome (PCOS) as it offers a wide range of benefits for those living with this condition. Regular physical activity can help regulate hormones, improve insulin sensitivity, and aid in weight management, all of which are key factors in managing PCOS symptoms. By incorporating exercise into your routine, you can take control of your health and experience significant improvements in your overall well-being.

One of the primary benefits of exercise for PCOS is its ability to regulate hormones. Hormonal imbalances are a common issue for women with PCOS, leading to irregular periods, acne, and unwanted hair growth. Exercise can help balance hormones by reducing levels of cortisol, the stress hormone, and increasing levels of serotonin, the feel-good hormone.

By regulating hormones through exercise, you can alleviate symptoms of PCOS and improve your quality of life.

In addition to hormone regulation, exercise has been shown to improve insulin sensitivity in women with PCOS. Insulin resistance is a common feature of PCOS, leading to high blood sugar levels and an increased risk of type 2 diabetes. Regular exercise can help combat insulin resistance by increasing the body's sensitivity to insulin, allowing for better control of blood sugar levels. By incorporating exercise into your routine, you can reduce the risk of developing diabetes and improve your overall metabolic health.

Another benefit of exercise for PCOS is its role in weight management. Many women with PCOS struggle with weight gain due to hormonal imbalances and insulin resistance. Regular physical activity can help control weight by burning calories, building muscle, and boosting metabolism. By incorporating exercise into your daily routine, you can achieve and maintain a healthy weight, reducing the risk of obesity-related complications and improving your overall health.

Overall, exercise is a powerful tool for managing PCOS naturally. By regulating hormones, improving insulin sensitivity, and aiding in weight management, exercise can help alleviate symptoms of PCOS and improve your overall well-being.

Incorporating regular physical activity into your routine can help you take control of your health and experience significant improvements in your PCOS symptoms. So lace up your sneakers, hit the gym, and start reaping the benefits of exercise for PCOS today.

Types of Exercise for PCOS

In order to effectively manage PCOS, incorporating regular exercise into your routine is crucial. There are various types of exercise that can help alleviate symptoms and improve overall health for women with PCOS. Understanding the different types of exercise and how they can benefit you is key to creating a personalized fitness plan that works for you.

One type of exercise that is highly recommended for women with PCOS is aerobic exercise. This type of exercise, also known as cardiovascular exercise, helps improve insulin sensitivity, which is often a concern for women with PCOS. Aerobic exercises like walking, running, cycling, and swimming can help regulate blood sugar levels, reduce inflammation, and aid in weight management.

Strength training is another important type of exercise for women with PCOS. Building muscle not only helps increase metabolism and burn more calories at rest, but it also helps improve insulin sensitivity. Incorporating strength training exercises like weightlifting, resistance band workouts, and bodyweight exercises can help build lean muscle mass and improve overall strength and endurance.

Yoga and Pilates are two types of exercise that can be particularly beneficial for women with PCOS. These mind-body practices focus on breath control, flexibility, and mindfulness, which can help reduce stress levels and improve hormonal balance. Both yoga and Pilates can help improve symptoms of PCOS such as irregular periods, acne, and weight gain.

High-intensity interval training (HIIT) is a type of exercise that involves short bursts of intense exercise followed by brief periods of rest or lower-intensity exercise. HIIT workouts can help improve cardiovascular fitness, burn more calories in less time, and improve insulin sensitivity.

Incorporating HIIT workouts into your fitness routine can help you see faster results and improve overall health.

Incorporating a combination of aerobic exercise, strength training, yoga, Pilates, and HIIT into your fitness routine can help you effectively manage PCOS symptoms and improve overall health.

It's important to consult with a healthcare provider or fitness professional before starting any new exercise program, especially if you have PCOS. Finding the right balance of exercise that works for you and fits into your lifestyle is key to healing PCOS naturally.

Creating an Exercise Routine

Creating an exercise routine is an essential component of managing and healing PCOS naturally. Regular physical activity has been shown to improve insulin sensitivity, reduce inflammation, and support weight management - all key factors in managing PCOS symptoms.

When creating an exercise routine, it's important to choose activities that you enjoy and that are sustainable for the long term. This will help you stay motivated and consistent with your workouts.

One of the best types of exercise for women with PCOS is strength training. Strength training helps build muscle mass, which can help improve insulin sensitivity and support weight loss.

It's also an effective way to boost your metabolism and increase your overall energy levels. Aim to incorporate strength training exercises at least two to three times per week, focusing on all major muscle groups.

In addition to strength training, cardiovascular exercise is also important for women with PCOS. Cardiovascular exercise helps improve heart health, boost mood, and support weight management. Aim to incorporate at least 150 minutes of moderate-intensity cardio per week, such as brisk walking, cycling, or swimming. You can also mix in high-intensity interval training (HIIT) for added benefits.

Flexibility and mobility exercises are also important components of an exercise routine for women with PCOS. Stretching and mobility work can help improve posture, reduce the risk of injury, and reduce muscle tension. Incorporate yoga, Pilates, or simple stretching routines into your weekly exercise plan to improve flexibility and mobility.

It's important to listen to your body and adjust your exercise routine as needed. If you're experiencing fatigue, pain, or other symptoms, it's important to rest and recover. Consult with a healthcare provider or a certified fitness professional to create a personalized exercise plan that aligns with your goals and abilities. Remember, consistency is key when it comes to creating an exercise routine that supports your PCOS healing journey.

Overcoming Barriers to Exercise

Exercise is a crucial component of managing PCOS naturally, but it can be difficult for many women with this condition to incorporate regular physical activity into their routines. There are several common barriers that may prevent individuals with PCOS from exercising regularly, but with some strategies and modifications, these obstacles can be overcome.

One of the most common barriers to exercise for women with PCOS is fatigue. Many individuals with PCOS experience chronic fatigue as a result of hormonal imbalances and other symptoms of the condition.

This can make it challenging to find the energy and motivation to exercise on a regular basis. To overcome this barrier, it can be helpful to start with low-impact activities such as walking or gentle yoga, and gradually increase the intensity as your energy levels improve.

Another common barrier to exercise for women with PCOS is pain. Many individuals with PCOS experience chronic pain, particularly in the pelvic area, which can make certain types of exercise uncomfortable or even impossible. To overcome this barrier, it may be helpful to work with a physical therapist or personal trainer who can help you modify exercises to reduce pain and discomfort. Additionally, incorporating activities such as swimming or cycling, which are easier on the joints, may be beneficial.

Time constraints are another major barrier to exercise for individuals with PCOS. Many women with this condition lead busy lives juggling work, family, and other responsibilities, leaving little time for physical activity. To overcome this barrier, it may be helpful to schedule exercise sessions into your calendar like any other appointment, and prioritize your health and well-being.

Additionally, incorporating short bursts of high-intensity exercise, such as interval training, can be an effective way to get a quick workout in when time is limited.

Mental health challenges, such as anxiety and depression, can also be significant barriers to exercise for women with PCOS. These conditions can make it difficult to find the motivation and energy to engage in physical activity, even though exercise has been shown to improve mood and reduce symptoms of anxiety and depression. To overcome this barrier, it may be helpful to seek support from a mental health professional, as well as incorporating mindfulness practices such as yoga or meditation into your exercise routine.

In conclusion, while there are many barriers to exercise for individuals with PCOS, there are also many strategies and modifications that can help overcome these obstacles. By starting with low-impact activities, modifying exercises to reduce pain and discomfort, scheduling exercise into your routine, and seeking support for mental health challenges, you can make physical activity a regular part of your life and experience the many benefits it has to offer in managing PCOS naturally. Remember that every step you take toward incorporating exercise into your life is a step toward healing and improving your overall health and well-being.

How To Heal PCOS Naturally

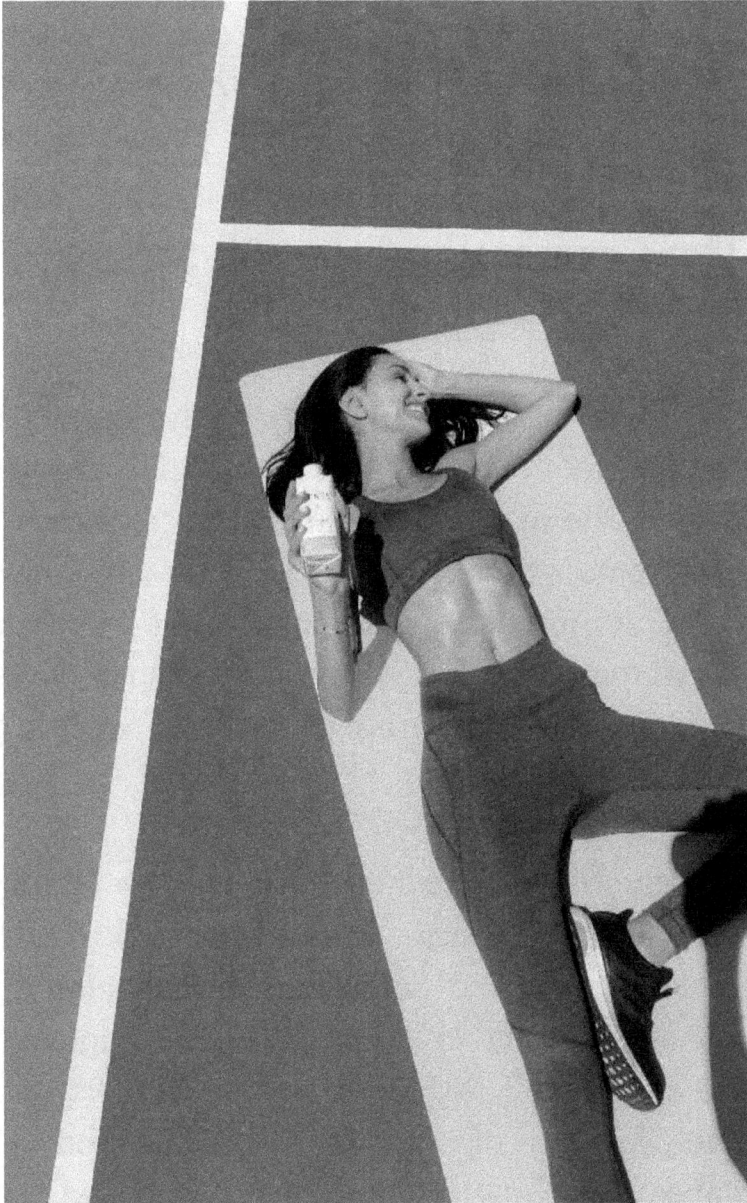

Chapter 4

Stress Management for PCOS

The Connection between Stress and PCOS

PCOS, or Polycystic Ovarian Syndrome, is a common hormonal disorder that affects many women worldwide. One of the key factors that can exacerbate the symptoms of PCOS is stress. Stress is known to have a direct impact on hormone levels in the body, and for women with PCOS, this can lead to an increase in symptoms such as irregular periods, weight gain, and difficulty conceiving.

Research has shown that women with PCOS who experience high levels of stress are more likely to have severe symptoms and complications associated with the condition. This is because stress triggers the release of cortisol, a hormone that can disrupt the delicate balance of hormones in the body. This imbalance can worsen symptoms of PCOS and make it harder for women to manage their condition effectively.

Managing stress is crucial for women with PCOS who are looking to heal their bodies naturally. By incorporating stress-reducing techniques such as meditation, yoga, deep breathing exercises, and regular physical activity into their daily routine, women with PCOS can help to rebalance their hormones and alleviate symptoms. Additionally, seeking support from a therapist or counselor can also be beneficial for women who are struggling to cope with the emotional toll of living with PCOS.

It is important for women with PCOS to recognize the connection between stress and their condition and take proactive steps to manage their stress levels effectively. By prioritizing self-care and incorporating stress-reducing techniques into their daily routine, women with PCOS can improve their overall health and well-being.

Ultimately, understanding and addressing the impact of stress on PCOS is a vital part of healing the body naturally and managing this complex hormonal disorder effectively.

Techniques for Reducing Stress

As someone living with Polycystic Ovarian Syndrome (PCOS), it is important to recognize the impact that stress can have on your overall health and well-being. Stress can exacerbate symptoms of PCOS such as irregular periods, acne, and weight gain.

In order to effectively manage your PCOS, it is essential to incorporate techniques for reducing stress into your daily routine.

One technique for reducing stress is practicing mindfulness and meditation. Taking time each day to quiet your mind and focus on the present moment can help alleviate feelings of anxiety and overwhelm. Deep breathing exercises can also be beneficial in calming the nervous system and reducing stress levels.

By incorporating these practices into your daily routine, you can cultivate a sense of inner peace and resilience in the face of stress.

Regular exercise is another powerful tool for reducing stress and managing PCOS symptoms. Physical activity releases endorphins, which are natural mood boosters that can help combat feelings of stress and anxiety. Exercise also helps regulate insulin levels and improve overall hormone balance, both of which are crucial for managing PCOS.

Whether it's going for a walk, practicing yoga, or hitting the gym, finding an exercise routine that you enjoy can be a game-changer in reducing stress and improving your overall health.

In addition to mindfulness, meditation, and exercise, it is important to prioritize self-care practices as a means of reducing stress. Taking time for yourself each day to engage in activities that bring you joy and relaxation can help replenish your energy reserves and build resilience to stress. Whether it's taking a warm bath, reading a book, or spending time in nature, finding ways to nurture yourself can have a profound impact on your mental and emotional well-being.

Finally, it is important to cultivate a supportive network of friends, family, and healthcare providers who can help you navigate the challenges of living with PCOS. Seeking out a counselor or therapist who specializes in women's health can also be beneficial in helping you develop coping strategies for managing stress.

By incorporating these techniques for reducing stress into your daily routine, you can empower yourself to take control of your PCOS and live a healthier, more balanced life.

Mindfulness and Meditation for PCOS

Mindfulness and meditation are powerful tools that can help women with PCOS manage their symptoms and improve their overall well-being. By practicing mindfulness, individuals can learn to be more present in the moment and better cope with the stress and anxiety that often accompany PCOS. This can help to reduce cortisol levels, which can have a positive impact on hormone balance and insulin resistance.

Meditation, on the other hand, can help women with PCOS connect with their bodies and minds on a deeper level. By taking time to quiet the mind and focus on breathing, individuals can reduce stress levels and promote relaxation. This can be particularly beneficial for women with PCOS, as stress can exacerbate symptoms and make it more difficult to manage the condition effectively.

Incorporating mindfulness and meditation into a daily routine can have a significant impact on PCOS symptoms. By taking just a few minutes each day to practice these techniques, individuals can reduce stress, improve hormone balance, and increase overall well-being. This can help to regulate menstrual cycles, reduce acne and hair growth, and improve fertility.

Mindfulness and meditation can also help women with PCOS make healthier lifestyle choices. By becoming more aware of their thoughts, feelings, and behaviors, individuals can better understand their triggers and make more conscious decisions about their diet, exercise, and self-care routines. This can help to reduce cravings, improve energy levels, and support weight management, all of which are important factors in managing PCOS.

Overall, incorporating mindfulness and meditation into a holistic approach to healing PCOS can have profound benefits for individuals struggling with this condition. By taking time each day to focus on the present moment and connect with their bodies and minds, women with PCOS can improve their symptoms, reduce stress, and promote overall well-being. These practices can be powerful tools in the journey to healing PCOS naturally.

Finding Balance in Your Life

Finding balance in your life is crucial when it comes to managing PCOS symptoms and promoting overall health and well-being. With the demands of work, family, and other responsibilities, it can be easy to neglect self-care and let stress take over. However, finding a balance between all aspects of your life is essential for managing PCOS naturally.

One way to find balance in your life is to prioritize self-care. This includes making time for activities that bring you joy and relaxation, such as exercise, meditation, or spending time with loved ones. Taking care of yourself is not selfish – it is necessary for managing PCOS and promoting overall health.

Another important aspect of finding balance in your life is managing stress. Stress can exacerbate PCOS symptoms and make it harder to manage the condition naturally. Finding healthy ways to cope with stress, such as practicing mindfulness or engaging in stress-reducing activities, can help you find balance and improve your overall well-being.

In addition to self-care and stress management, finding balance in your life also involves making healthy lifestyle choices. This includes eating a balanced diet, getting regular exercise, and prioritizing sleep. These lifestyle choices can help manage PCOS symptoms and improve your overall health and well-being.

Overall, finding balance in your life is essential for managing PCOS naturally. By prioritizing self-care, managing stress, and making healthy lifestyle choices, you can take control of your health and well-being. Remember, it is important to listen to your body and make choices that support your overall health and happiness.

How To Heal PCOS Naturally

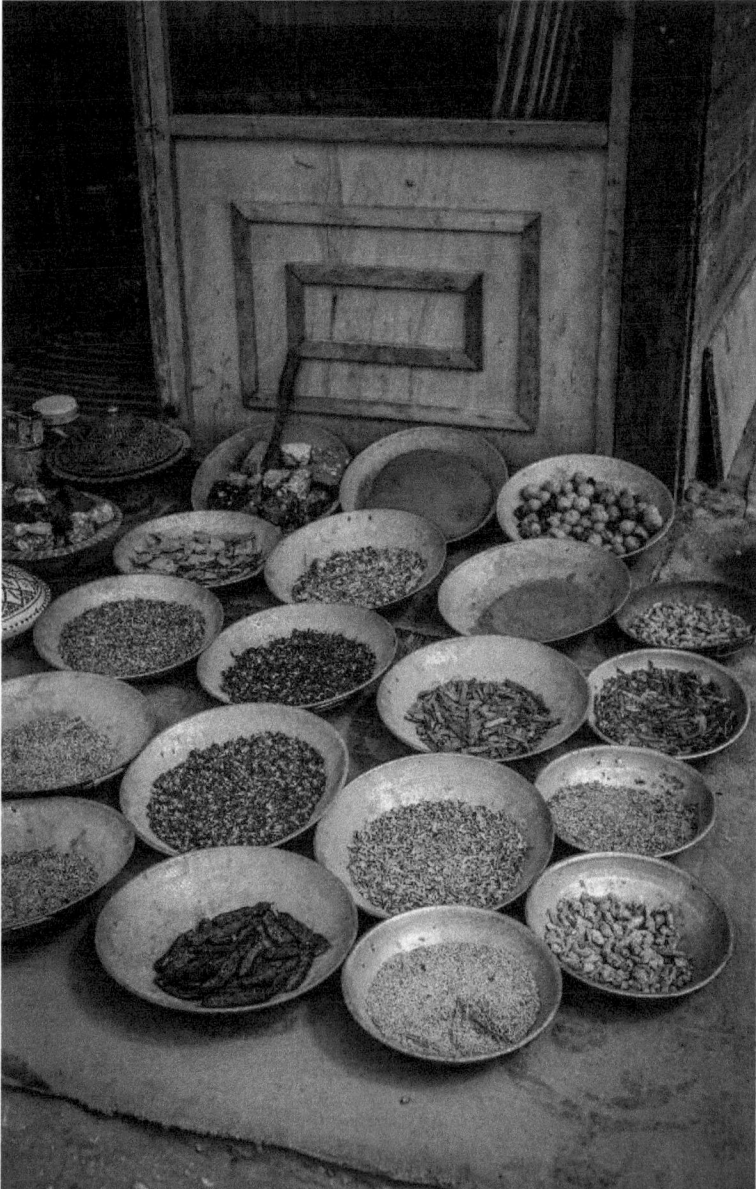

A Comprehensive Guide for Women

Chapter 5

Natural Supplements for PCOS

Vitamins and Minerals for PCOS

Having PCOS can be challenging, but there are natural ways to manage its symptoms and improve your overall health. One important aspect of managing PCOS is ensuring you are getting the right vitamins and minerals in your diet. In this subchapter, we will explore the essential vitamins and minerals that can help support your body in managing PCOS effectively.

One key vitamin for women with PCOS is vitamin D. Research has shown that many women with PCOS have lower levels of vitamin D, which can contribute to insulin resistance and other symptoms of the condition. It is important to get your vitamin D levels checked and to consider supplementing if necessary. Vitamin D can also help regulate menstrual cycles and support overall reproductive health.

Another important vitamin for women with PCOS is B vitamins, particularly B6 and B12. B vitamins play a crucial role in hormone regulation and can help support energy levels and mood. Ensuring you are getting enough B vitamins in your diet or through supplementation can help alleviate some of the symptoms of PCOS, such as fatigue and mood swings.

In addition to vitamins, certain minerals are also important for women with PCOS. One mineral that is particularly beneficial is magnesium. Magnesium can help regulate blood sugar levels, support hormone balance, and reduce inflammation in the body. Including magnesium-rich foods in your diet, such as leafy greens, nuts, and seeds, can be beneficial for managing PCOS symptoms.

Overall, incorporating a variety of vitamins and minerals into your diet can help support your body in managing PCOS naturally. It is important to work with a healthcare provider or a nutritionist to determine the right supplements for your individual needs. By focusing on nutrient-dense foods and ensuring you are meeting your body's nutritional needs, you can take steps towards healing PCOS naturally and improving your overall well-being.

Herbal Supplements for PCOS

If you have PCOS, you may have tried various medications and treatments to manage your symptoms. However, you may not be aware of the potential benefits of incorporating herbal supplements into your treatment plan. Herbal supplements can be a natural and effective way to help manage the symptoms of PCOS and promote overall well-being.

One popular herbal supplement for PCOS is chasteberry, also known as Vitex. Chasteberry has been used for centuries to help regulate menstrual cycles and hormone levels. Studies have shown that chasteberry can help reduce symptoms such as irregular periods, acne, and hirsutism in women with PCOS. It works by balancing levels of the hormone prolactin, which can be elevated in women with PCOS.

Another herbal supplement that may be beneficial for women with PCOS is cinnamon. Cinnamon has been shown to help regulate blood sugar levels, which is important for women with PCOS who may have insulin resistance. By helping to control blood sugar levels, cinnamon may also help reduce symptoms such as weight gain and cravings for sugary foods.

Milk thistle is another herbal supplement that may be helpful for women with PCOS. Milk thistle is known for its liver-protective properties and may help support liver function in women with PCOS, who may be more prone to liver issues due to insulin resistance.

A healthy liver is essential for hormone balance and overall health, so incorporating milk thistle into your treatment plan may be beneficial.

In addition to these herbal supplements, it's important to remember that diet and lifestyle changes are also key components of managing PCOS naturally. Eating a balanced diet rich in whole foods, staying active, and managing stress levels are all important for managing PCOS symptoms.

By incorporating herbal supplements along with these healthy lifestyle changes, you may be able to effectively manage your PCOS and improve your overall health and well-being.

Incorporating Supplements into Your Routine

Incorporating supplements into your routine can be a powerful tool in managing and healing PCOS naturally. While a healthy diet and lifestyle are essential components of managing this condition, supplements can provide additional support to address specific symptoms and imbalances associated with PCOS. By working with a healthcare provider or nutritionist, you can create a personalized supplement plan that is tailored to your individual needs.

One of the most commonly recommended supplements for PCOS is inositol, a type of B vitamin that has been shown to improve insulin sensitivity and regulate menstrual cycles. Inositol can be particularly beneficial for women with PCOS who struggle with insulin resistance, as it can help to lower blood sugar levels and reduce the risk of developing type 2 diabetes. Other supplements that may be helpful for managing PCOS include omega-3 fatty acids, which can help to reduce inflammation and improve hormone balance, and magnesium, which can help to support energy production and reduce stress.

When incorporating supplements into your routine, it is important to start slowly and monitor how your body responds. Some supplements may cause digestive upset or interact with medications you are taking, so it is important to consult with a healthcare provider before adding any new supplements to your regimen. It is also important to choose high-quality supplements from reputable brands to ensure that you are getting the most benefit from your supplementation.

In addition to taking supplements, it is important to focus on other aspects of your health such as diet, exercise, and stress management. Supplements should be viewed as a complement to these lifestyle changes, rather than a replacement for them. By taking a holistic approach to managing your PCOS, you can address the root causes of your symptoms and improve your overall health and well-being.

Overall, incorporating supplements into your routine can be a valuable tool in managing and healing PCOS naturally.

By working with a healthcare provider or nutritionist to create a personalized supplement plan, you can address specific symptoms and imbalances associated with PCOS and support your overall health and well-being. With the right combination of supplements, diet, exercise, and stress management, you can take control of your PCOS and experience improved quality of life.

Potential Risks and Side Effects

Living with Polycystic Ovarian Syndrome (PCOS) can be challenging, as it comes with a host of potential risks and side effects that can impact a woman's quality of life. It is important for individuals with PCOS to be aware of these risks in order to properly manage their condition and prevent any further complications.

One of the main risks associated with PCOS is infertility. Many women with PCOS struggle to conceive due to irregular ovulation and hormone imbalances. This can be a devastating side effect for those who hope to start a family.

However, there are natural ways to improve fertility in women with PCOS, such as maintaining a healthy weight, managing stress levels, and incorporating fertility-boosting foods into their diet.

Another potential risk of PCOS is an increased risk of developing type 2 diabetes. Insulin resistance is a common characteristic of PCOS, which can lead to high blood sugar levels and eventually diabetes if left unmanaged. It is important for individuals with PCOS to monitor their blood sugar levels regularly and adopt a healthy lifestyle that includes regular exercise and a balanced diet to reduce their risk of developing diabetes.

In addition to infertility and diabetes, women with PCOS are also at a higher risk of developing other health conditions such as heart disease, high blood pressure, and endometrial cancer. These risks highlight the importance of taking proactive steps to manage PCOS and reduce the likelihood of experiencing these serious health complications.

By making healthy lifestyle choices, such as eating a nutritious diet, staying physically active, and managing stress, individuals with PCOS can improve their overall health and reduce their risk of developing these conditions.

In conclusion, understanding the potential risks and side effects of PCOS is essential for individuals who are living with this condition. By being aware of these risks, individuals can take proactive steps to manage their PCOS effectively and reduce their risk of developing further complications. With the right lifestyle changes and support from healthcare professionals, women with PCOS can improve their overall health and well-being and live a fulfilling life despite their condition.

How To Heal PCOS Naturally

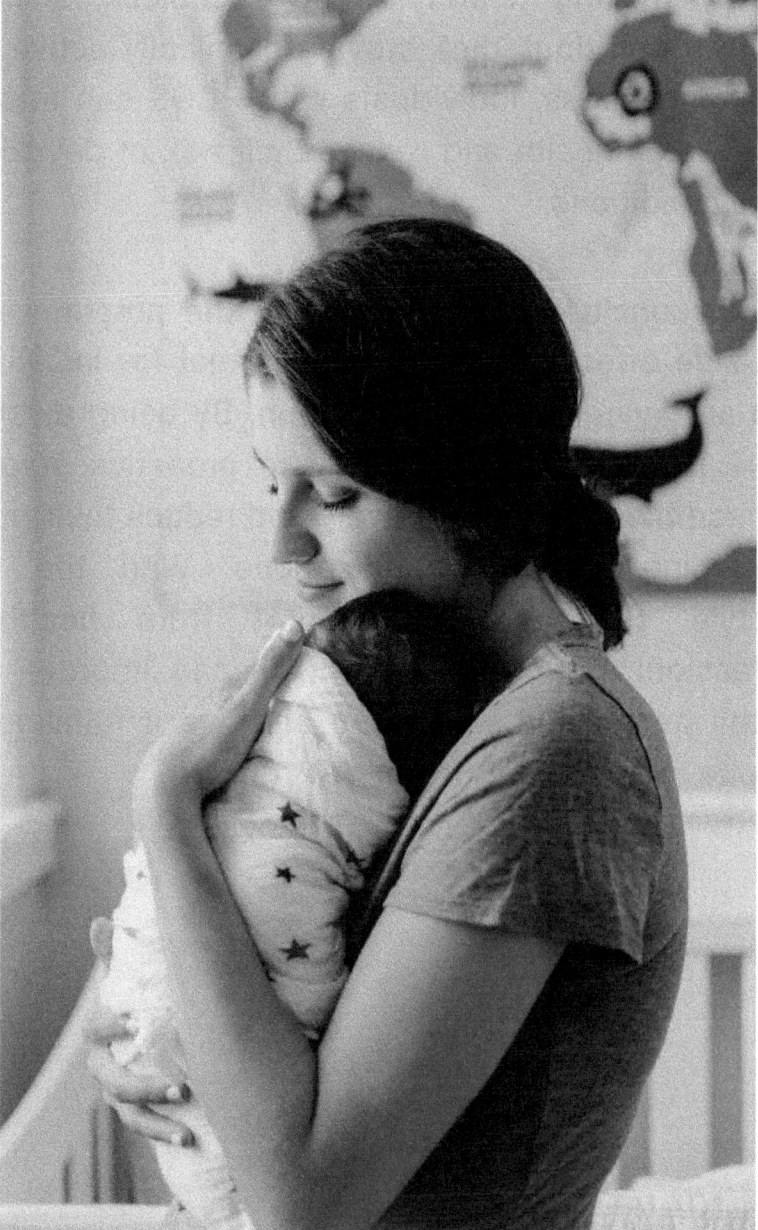

A Comprehensive Guide for Women

Chapter 6

Fertility and PCOS

Understanding Fertility and PCOS

One of the most common concerns for women with PCOS is difficulty getting pregnant. PCOS can have a significant impact on fertility due to hormonal imbalances and irregular menstrual cycles. It is important for women with PCOS to understand how their condition affects their fertility in order to make informed decisions about their reproductive health.

Women with PCOS often have higher levels of androgens, such as testosterone, which can interfere with ovulation and the ability to conceive. Additionally, insulin resistance, a common symptom of PCOS, can also contribute to fertility issues by disrupting hormone levels and affecting egg development. These factors can make it more challenging for women with PCOS to get pregnant, but there are natural ways to improve fertility and increase the chances of conceiving.

One key aspect of managing fertility with PCOS is maintaining a healthy lifestyle. This includes eating a balanced diet, exercising regularly, and managing stress levels. By reducing inflammation in the body and balancing hormone levels, women with PCOS can improve their fertility and increase their chances of conceiving. Additionally, certain supplements and herbs can help regulate menstrual cycles and support ovulation, further improving fertility outcomes.

It is also important for women with PCOS to work closely with a healthcare provider or fertility specialist to address any underlying issues that may be affecting fertility.

By monitoring hormone levels, tracking ovulation, and exploring treatment options such as medication or assisted reproductive technologies, women with PCOS can take proactive steps to improve their fertility and increase their chances of conceiving. With the right support and guidance, women with PCOS can achieve their goal of starting a family naturally.

Overall, understanding fertility and PCOS is essential for women with this condition who are hoping to conceive. By taking a holistic approach to managing PCOS through lifestyle changes, supplements, and working with healthcare professionals, women with PCOS can optimize their fertility and increase their chances of getting pregnant. With patience, perseverance, and the right tools, women with PCOS can overcome fertility challenges and achieve their dream of starting a family.

Options for Fertility Treatments

For women with PCOS who are struggling with infertility, there are several options available to help increase the chances of conceiving. One common treatment is ovulation induction, which involves taking medication to stimulate the ovaries to release eggs.

This can help regulate the menstrual cycle and improve the chances of getting pregnant. Another option is intrauterine insemination (IUI), where sperm is directly inserted into the uterus to increase the chances of fertilization.

In vitro fertilization (IVF) is another option for women with PCOS who are having trouble getting pregnant. This procedure involves retrieving eggs from the ovaries, fertilizing them with sperm in a lab, and then transferring the embryos into the uterus. IVF can be a more invasive and expensive option, but it can also be very effective for women with PCOS.

Some women with PCOS may benefit from lifestyle changes and natural treatments to improve their fertility. Eating a healthy diet, exercising regularly, and managing stress can all help regulate hormone levels and improve the chances of conceiving. There are also natural supplements and herbs that can help support fertility, such as vitex, maca, and inositol.

Acupuncture and traditional Chinese medicine (TCM) are also popular options for women with PCOS who are trying to conceive. Acupuncture can help regulate hormone levels, improve blood flow to the reproductive organs, and reduce stress, all of which can improve fertility. TCM practitioners may also recommend herbal remedies and dietary changes to support fertility.

Ultimately, the best fertility treatment for women with PCOS will depend on their individual circumstances and goals. It's important to work with a healthcare provider who specializes in PCOS and fertility to develop a personalized treatment plan that addresses your unique needs. By exploring all of the options available and taking a holistic approach to healing PCOS naturally, women can increase their chances of conceiving and starting a family.

Tips for Improving Fertility with PCOS

If you have been diagnosed with Polycystic Ovary Syndrome (PCOS) and are struggling to conceive, there are several natural ways you can improve your fertility. In this subchapter, we will discuss some tips for improving fertility with PCOS that can help you on your journey to becoming a mother.

One of the most important things you can do to improve your fertility with PCOS is to maintain a healthy weight. Research has shown that even a modest weight loss of 5-10% can help regulate your menstrual cycles and improve your chances of conceiving. Eating a balanced diet rich in fruits, vegetables, whole grains, and lean proteins can help you achieve and maintain a healthy weight.

Exercise is another key factor in improving fertility with PCOS. Regular physical activity can help reduce insulin resistance, regulate your menstrual cycles, and improve your overall health. Aim for at least 30 minutes of moderate exercise, such as brisk walking or cycling, most days of the week to help improve your fertility.

Managing stress is also important for improving fertility with PCOS. Chronic stress can disrupt hormone levels and make it more difficult to conceive. Practicing relaxation techniques such as deep breathing, meditation, or yoga can help reduce stress and improve your fertility. It is also important to get an adequate amount of sleep each night to support your overall health and fertility.

In addition to these lifestyle factors, certain supplements and herbs may also help improve fertility with PCOS. Inositol, a type of B vitamin, has been shown to improve insulin sensitivity and regulate menstrual cycles in women with PCOS.

Other supplements such as omega-3 fatty acids, vitamin D, and magnesium may also support fertility. Consulting with a healthcare provider or a naturopathic doctor can help you determine which supplements are right for you.

By making these lifestyle changes and incorporating supplements and herbs into your routine, you can improve your fertility and increase your chances of conceiving with PCOS. Remember to be patient and gentle with yourself as you navigate this journey, and seek support from healthcare providers, friends, and family members who can help you along the way. With dedication and perseverance, you can improve your fertility and achieve your dream of becoming a mother.

Support for Women Trying to Conceive with PCOS

For women with Polycystic Ovarian Syndrome (PCOS) who are trying to conceive, the journey can often be filled with challenges and obstacles. However, it is important to remember that there is hope and support available for those who are struggling to become pregnant. One of the first steps in seeking support for infertility related to PCOS is to find a healthcare provider who is knowledgeable about the condition and can offer guidance and treatment options tailored to your specific needs.

In addition to medical support, many women find comfort and encouragement through support groups and online communities dedicated to PCOS and fertility issues. These groups can provide a safe space to share experiences, ask questions, and receive emotional support from others who are going through similar struggles. Connecting with others who understand what you are going through can help alleviate feelings of isolation and provide a sense of community during this challenging time.

Another important aspect of supporting women with PCOS who are trying to conceive is to focus on lifestyle changes that can improve fertility and overall health. This may include following a healthy diet rich in whole foods, engaging in regular exercise, managing stress levels, and getting enough sleep.

Making these lifestyle changes can not only improve your chances of conceiving but also help manage symptoms of PCOS and promote overall well-being.

For women who are struggling with infertility related to PCOS, there are also various treatment options available that can help increase their chances of conceiving. These may include medications to regulate ovulation, assisted reproductive technologies such as in vitro fertilization (IVF), or surgical interventions to address underlying issues such as ovarian cysts or hormonal imbalances.

It is important to work closely with your healthcare provider to determine the best course of treatment for your individual needs and preferences.

Overall, it is essential for women with PCOS who are trying to conceive to seek out the support and resources they need to navigate this challenging journey. By finding a healthcare provider who understands their unique needs, connecting with others who can offer emotional support, making lifestyle changes to promote fertility and overall health, and exploring treatment options tailored to their individual circumstances, women with PCOS can increase their chances of achieving their dream of becoming parents. Remember, you are not alone in this journey, and there is support available to help you every step of the way.

How To Heal PCOS Naturally

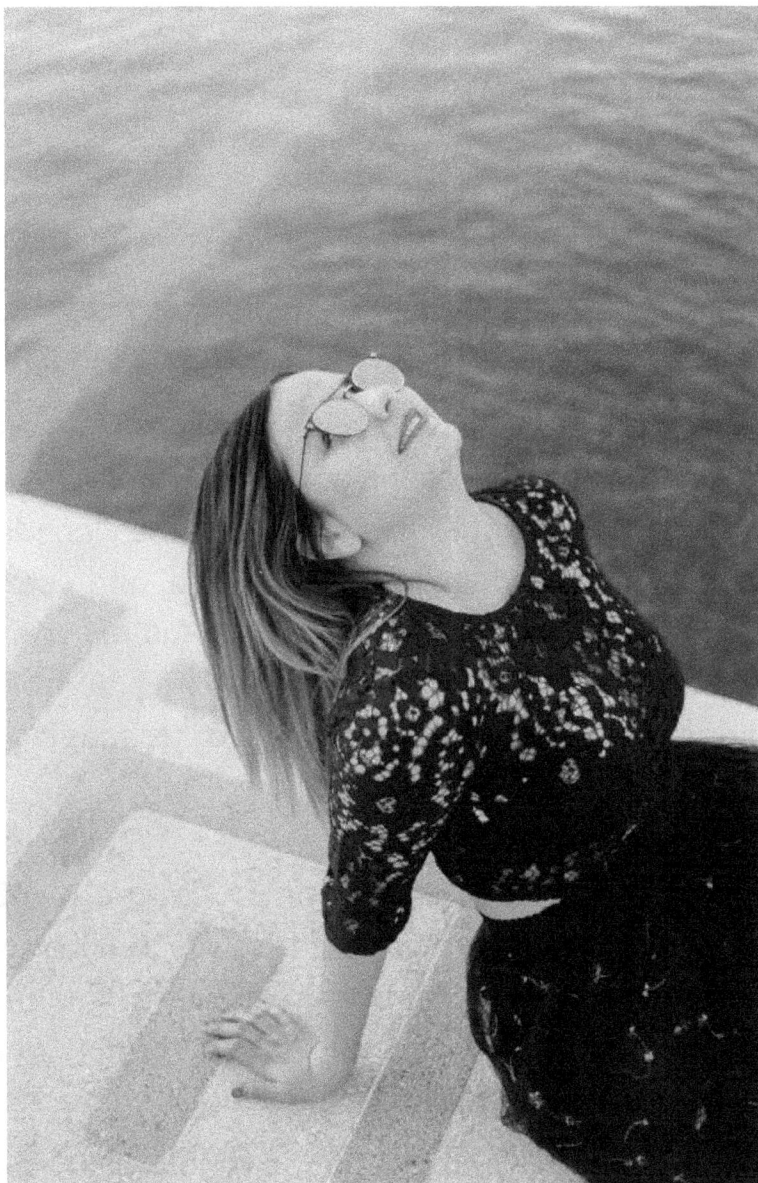

A Comprehensive Guide for Women

Chapter 7

Hormone Balance and PCOS

The Role of Hormones in PCOS

In women with Polycystic Ovary Syndrome (PCOS), hormones play a crucial role in the development and progression of the condition. Hormones such as insulin, testosterone, and estrogen can all have an impact on the symptoms experienced by women with PCOS. Understanding the role of hormones in PCOS is essential for managing the condition effectively and naturally.

Insulin resistance is a common feature of PCOS, where the body's cells become less responsive to the hormone insulin. This can lead to elevated blood sugar levels, weight gain, and increased production of testosterone. High levels of insulin can stimulate the ovaries to produce more testosterone, which can disrupt the menstrual cycle and lead to symptoms such as acne, hair loss, and irregular periods.

Managing insulin levels through diet, exercise, and lifestyle changes can help improve symptoms and restore hormone balance in women with PCOS.

Testosterone is a male hormone that is also present in women, but elevated levels of testosterone in women with PCOS can lead to symptoms such as hirsutism (excessive hair growth), acne, and male-pattern baldness. High levels of testosterone can disrupt the menstrual cycle and interfere with ovulation, making it difficult for women with PCOS to conceive. Balancing testosterone levels through diet, exercise, and natural supplements can help alleviate symptoms and improve fertility in women with PCOS.

Estrogen is a female hormone that plays a key role in regulating the menstrual cycle and promoting ovulation. Women with PCOS may have imbalances in estrogen levels, which can lead to irregular periods, anovulation, and fertility issues. Estrogen dominance, where there is an excess of estrogen relative to progesterone, can contribute to symptoms such as heavy periods, bloating, and mood swings. Supporting estrogen metabolism through diet, lifestyle changes, and natural therapies can help restore hormone balance and improve symptoms in women with PCOS.

In conclusion, hormones play a significant role in the development and progression of PCOS. Understanding how hormones such as insulin, testosterone, and estrogen interact in the body can help women with PCOS manage their symptoms and improve their overall health.

By addressing hormone imbalances through diet, exercise, and natural therapies, women with PCOS can heal their bodies naturally and achieve optimal hormone balance. Taking a holistic approach to healing PCOS can lead to long-lasting improvements in symptoms and overall well-being for women with this complex hormonal condition.

Natural Ways to Balance Hormones

Balancing hormones is essential for managing PCOS symptoms and promoting overall health and well-being. Fortunately, there are natural ways to help restore hormonal balance and alleviate the symptoms of PCOS. By incorporating these strategies into your daily routine, you can take control of your health and empower yourself on your healing journey.

One of the most effective ways to balance hormones naturally is through diet. Consuming a balanced diet rich in whole, nutrient-dense foods can help regulate insulin levels, reduce inflammation, and support hormonal balance.

Focus on incorporating plenty of fruits, vegetables, lean proteins, and healthy fats into your meals, while limiting processed foods, sugar, and refined carbohydrates. Eating a well-rounded diet can help stabilize blood sugar levels, which is crucial for managing insulin resistance, a common issue in women with PCOS.

Regular exercise is another powerful tool for balancing hormones and managing PCOS symptoms. Physical activity can help regulate insulin levels, reduce inflammation, and support healthy hormone production. Aim for at least 30 minutes of moderate exercise most days of the week, such as walking, cycling, or yoga. Find activities that you enjoy and make them a regular part of your routine to support hormonal balance and overall well-being.

Stress management is also key to balancing hormones naturally. Chronic stress can disrupt hormone levels and exacerbate PCOS symptoms. Incorporating relaxation techniques such as deep breathing, meditation, or mindfulness can help reduce stress levels and support hormonal balance. Prioritize self-care practices that help you relax and unwind, such as taking a warm bath, reading a book, or spending time in nature. By managing stress effectively, you can support your body's ability to balance hormones and promote healing.

In addition to diet, exercise, and stress management, there are several natural supplements that can help support hormonal balance in women with PCOS. Supplements such as omega-3 fatty acids, magnesium, and vitamin D have been shown to support hormone production, reduce inflammation, and improve insulin sensitivity. Consult with a healthcare provider or naturopath to determine which supplements may be beneficial for you and to ensure they are safe and appropriate for your individual needs. By incorporating these natural strategies into your daily routine, you can take proactive steps to balance hormones, manage PCOS symptoms, and support your overall health and well-being.

Managing Symptoms through Hormone Regulation

Managing symptoms through hormone regulation is a crucial aspect of finding relief from Polycystic Ovary Syndrome (PCOS). One of the key hormones that play a significant role in PCOS is insulin. Insulin resistance is common in women with PCOS, leading to high levels of insulin in the blood. This can contribute to weight gain, high blood sugar levels, and increased production of androgens, the male hormones that are elevated in PCOS. By regulating insulin levels through dietary changes and exercise, women with PCOS can help manage their symptoms and improve their overall health.

Another important hormone to consider in managing PCOS symptoms is cortisol, the stress hormone. High levels of stress can exacerbate PCOS symptoms, leading to increased inflammation, weight gain, and hormonal imbalances. Finding ways to reduce stress through practices such as meditation, yoga, or deep breathing exercises can help regulate cortisol levels and improve symptoms of PCOS.

Additionally, getting an adequate amount of sleep and practicing good sleep hygiene can also help regulate cortisol levels and improve overall hormone balance.

Balancing estrogen and progesterone levels is another important aspect of managing PCOS symptoms. Women with PCOS often have imbalances in these hormones, leading to irregular menstrual cycles, infertility, and other symptoms.

By incorporating foods rich in phytoestrogens, such as flaxseeds, soy, and legumes, into their diet, women with PCOS can help regulate estrogen levels. Additionally, herbs such as chasteberry and black cohosh can help regulate progesterone levels and promote hormonal balance.

In addition to dietary changes and stress management techniques, incorporating regular exercise into your routine can also help regulate hormones and manage PCOS symptoms.

Exercise has been shown to improve insulin sensitivity, reduce inflammation, and promote weight loss, all of which can help alleviate symptoms of PCOS. Aim for a combination of cardiovascular exercise, strength training, and flexibility exercises to support overall health and hormone regulation.

By focusing on hormone regulation through dietary changes, stress management, and regular exercise, women with PCOS can take control of their symptoms and improve their overall health and well-being.

It's important to work with a healthcare provider or a qualified nutritionist to develop a personalized plan that addresses your specific needs and goals. With dedication and consistency, managing PCOS symptoms through hormone regulation is possible, allowing women to heal naturally and live a healthier, happier life.

Working with Healthcare Providers to Address Hormone Imbalance

Having PCOS can be overwhelming, but working with healthcare providers is essential in addressing hormone imbalances. It's important to find a healthcare provider who understands PCOS and is willing to work with you to find natural solutions.

This subchapter will provide guidance on how to effectively communicate with your healthcare provider and collaborate on a treatment plan that works for you.

First and foremost, it's important to find a healthcare provider who specializes in treating PCOS. This could be an endocrinologist, gynecologist, or a naturopathic doctor who has experience in treating hormonal imbalances.

Make sure to do your research and ask for recommendations from other women with PCOS. Once you have found a provider, schedule an appointment to discuss your symptoms and concerns.

During your appointment, be open and honest about your symptoms and how they are impacting your daily life. It's important to communicate your goals and desires for treatment, whether that includes natural remedies, lifestyle changes, or medication. Your healthcare provider should listen to your concerns and work with you to create a personalized treatment plan that addresses your hormone imbalances.

In addition to communicating with your healthcare provider, it's important to be proactive in your own health journey. This may include keeping a journal of your symptoms, tracking your menstrual cycle, and making note of any changes in your diet or lifestyle.

By being actively involved in your treatment plan, you can better understand how certain interventions are affecting your hormone levels and overall health.

Remember, healing PCOS naturally is a journey that requires patience and dedication. Working with a healthcare provider who understands your unique needs and concerns is key in addressing hormone imbalances. By being proactive and open in your communication, you can work together to find solutions that help you achieve hormonal balance and improve your quality of life.

How To Heal PCOS Naturally

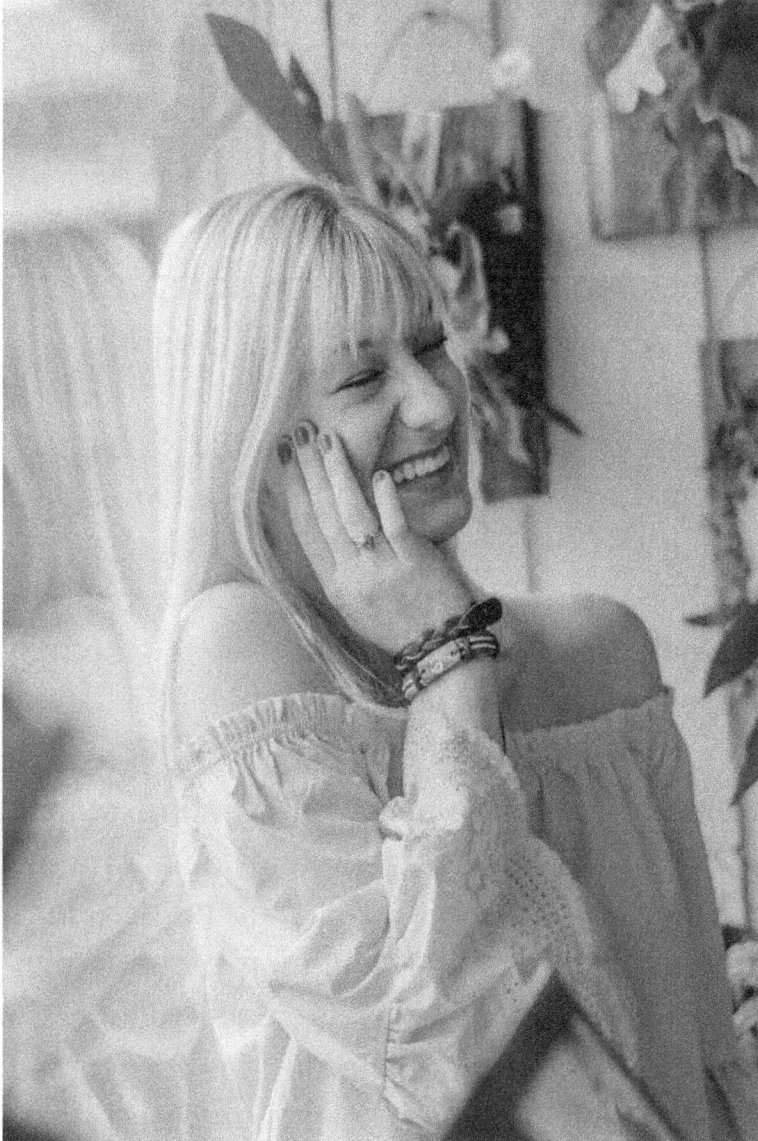

Chapter 8

Lifestyle Changes for Long-Term Healing

Creating Sustainable Habits for PCOS Management

Creating sustainable habits for PCOS management is crucial for long-term success in managing the symptoms of this condition. By making small changes to your daily routine, you can improve your overall health and well-being while also reducing the impact of PCOS on your life.

One of the first steps in creating sustainable habits for PCOS management is to focus on a healthy diet. Eating a balanced diet that is rich in fruits, vegetables, whole grains, and lean proteins can help regulate blood sugar levels and reduce insulin resistance, which are common issues for women with PCOS. Avoiding processed foods, sugary drinks, and high-fat foods can also help improve your symptoms and overall health.

In addition to eating a healthy diet, regular exercise is essential for managing PCOS symptoms. Physical activity can help improve insulin sensitivity, regulate hormone levels, and promote weight loss, all of which can help alleviate the symptoms of PCOS. Aim for at least 30 minutes of moderate exercise most days of the week, such as walking, biking, or swimming, to help manage your PCOS symptoms.

Stress management is another important aspect of creating sustainable habits for PCOS management. High levels of stress can exacerbate PCOS symptoms and make it more difficult to manage the condition. Incorporating stress-reducing activities into your daily routine, such as yoga, meditation, deep breathing exercises, or spending time in nature, can help improve your overall well-being and reduce the impact of stress on your PCOS symptoms.

Lastly, getting enough sleep is crucial for managing PCOS symptoms and overall health. Poor sleep can disrupt hormone levels, increase insulin resistance, and worsen PCOS symptoms.

Aim for 7-9 hours of quality sleep each night by establishing a bedtime routine, creating a relaxing sleep environment, and avoiding caffeine and electronics before bed. By incorporating these sustainable habits into your daily routine, you can effectively manage your PCOS symptoms and improve your overall health and well-being.

Setting Realistic Goals for Healing

Setting realistic goals for healing is an important step in managing PCOS naturally. Many people with PCOS may feel overwhelmed by the prospect of making significant lifestyle changes, but breaking down your goals into smaller, more achievable steps can help you stay motivated and on track. By setting realistic goals, you can gradually make positive changes that will support your overall health and well-being.

When setting goals for healing, it's important to consider your individual needs and limitations. Every person with PCOS is different, and what works for one person may not work for another.

Take the time to assess your current health and lifestyle habits, and identify areas where you can make improvements. Set specific, measurable goals that are tailored to your unique situation, and be realistic about what you can achieve in a given timeframe.

One helpful strategy for setting realistic goals is to focus on making small, sustainable changes. Instead of trying to overhaul your entire lifestyle overnight, start by making one or two small changes at a time. This could be as simple as adding more fruits and vegetables to your diet, or committing to a regular exercise routine. By making gradual changes, you can build healthy habits that will support your long-term health and well-being.

It's also important to track your progress as you work towards your healing goals. Keeping a journal or using a tracking app can help you stay accountable and motivated, and allow you to see how far you've come. Celebrate your successes, no matter how small, and be kind to yourself if you experience setbacks. Healing is a journey, and it's important to be patient and compassionate with yourself as you work towards your goals.

Ultimately, setting realistic goals for healing is about taking control of your health and well-being. By breaking down your goals into manageable steps, focusing on sustainable changes, and tracking your progress, you can make positive changes that will support your overall health and well-being. Remember that healing is a journey, and it's okay to take things one step at a time. With dedication and perseverance, you can make positive changes that will help you manage your PCOS naturally and improve your quality of life.

Tracking Progress and Adjusting as Needed

Tracking progress and adjusting as needed are crucial components in the journey to healing PCOS naturally. By monitoring your symptoms, lifestyle changes, and treatment protocols, you can gain valuable insights into what is working for you and what may need to be adjusted. This proactive approach empowers you to take control of your health and make informed decisions that will lead to improved outcomes.

One effective way to track your progress is by keeping a symptom journal. This can help you identify patterns and triggers that may be exacerbating your symptoms. By recording details such as your menstrual cycles, energy levels, mood, and any changes in diet or exercise, you can start to see correlations between certain behaviors and your PCOS symptoms. This information can then be used to make targeted adjustments to your lifestyle or treatment plan.

Another important aspect of tracking progress is regularly monitoring key markers such as hormone levels, insulin resistance, and weight. This can be done through blood tests, hormonal panels, or other diagnostic tests recommended by your healthcare provider.

By tracking these markers over time, you can see how your body is responding to your natural healing protocols and make adjustments as needed to optimize your results.

It's important to remember that healing PCOS naturally is a journey, not a quick fix. Progress may be gradual, and setbacks may occur along the way. By adopting a mindset of patience and perseverance, you can stay focused on your goals and continue making progress towards improved health and well-being. Remember to celebrate your successes, no matter how small, and use any setbacks as learning opportunities to make necessary adjustments and keep moving forward.

In conclusion, tracking progress and adjusting as needed are essential strategies for healing PCOS naturally. By staying informed, proactive, and patient, you can empower yourself to take control of your health and make meaningful changes that will lead to improved outcomes.

Remember that every step you take towards healing is a step in the right direction, and with dedication and perseverance, you can achieve lasting health and wellness.

Building a Support System for Continued Success

In order to effectively manage and heal PCOS naturally, it is crucial to establish a strong support system. Dealing with the symptoms and challenges of PCOS can be overwhelming at times, and having a network of people who understand and support you can make all the difference. Whether it's family, friends, or a support group of fellow PCOS warriors, having a group of people who can offer encouragement, advice, and understanding can help you stay motivated and on track with your healing journey.

One key aspect of building a support system for continued success is finding healthcare providers who are knowledgeable about PCOS and are supportive of natural healing methods. This may involve seeking out holistic practitioners, naturopathic doctors, or functional medicine specialists who can provide guidance and support in your healing journey.

These healthcare providers can help you develop a personalized treatment plan that addresses the root causes of your PCOS and incorporates natural therapies such as dietary changes, supplements, and lifestyle modifications.

In addition to healthcare providers, it is important to surround yourself with a supportive community of like-minded individuals who are also on a journey to heal PCOS naturally. This may involve joining online support groups, attending local meetups, or participating in workshops and events focused on PCOS and natural healing. Connecting with others who are going through similar challenges can provide a sense of camaraderie and solidarity, as well as valuable tips and resources for managing PCOS naturally.

Building a support system for continued success also involves taking care of your mental and emotional well-being. Living with a chronic condition like PCOS can be emotionally taxing, and it's important to prioritize self-care practices that promote mental and emotional resilience.

This may include practices such as mindfulness meditation, journaling, therapy, or engaging in activities that bring you joy and relaxation. By taking care of your mental and emotional health, you can better cope with the challenges of PCOS and stay focused on your healing journey.

Ultimately, building a strong support system for continued success in healing PCOS naturally involves surrounding yourself with people who believe in your ability to heal and thrive. By cultivating a network of supportive individuals, healthcare providers, and self-care practices, you can create a foundation of strength and resilience that will empower you to overcome the challenges of PCOS and live a vibrant, healthy life.

Remember, you are not alone in your healing journey, and with the right support system in place, you can achieve lasting success in managing and healing PCOS naturally.

How To Heal PCOS Naturally

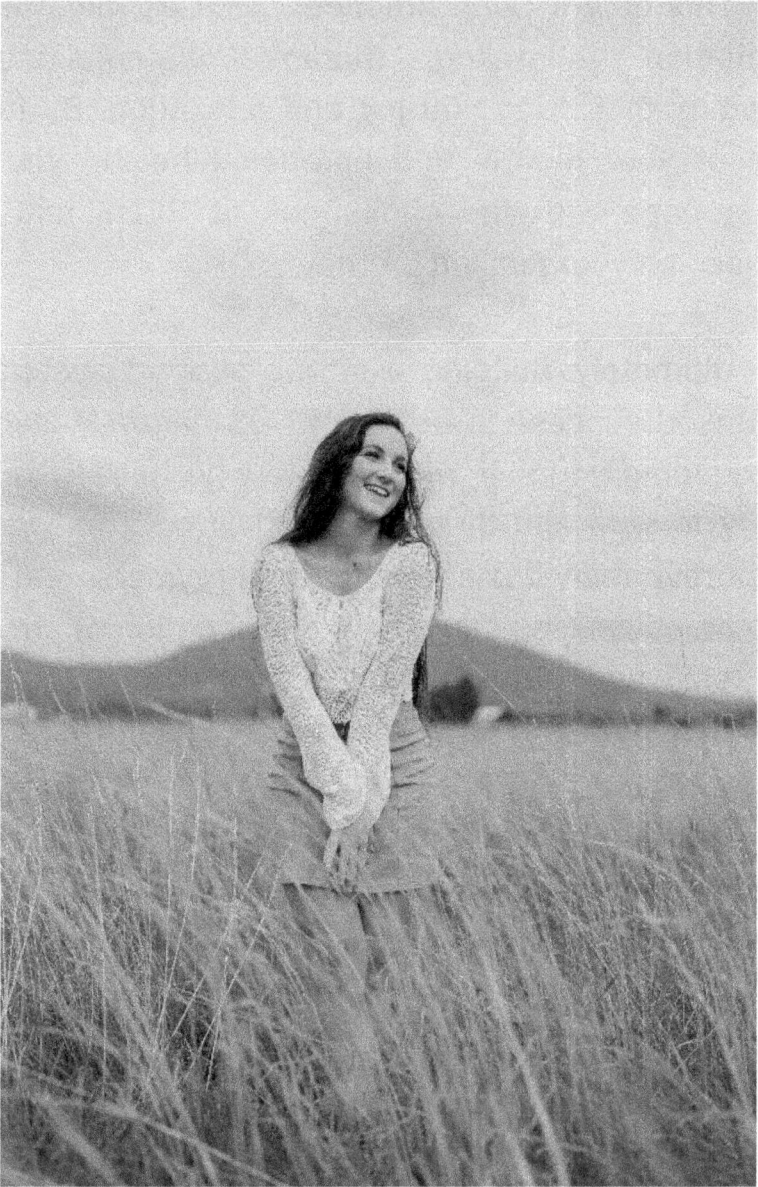

Chapter 9

Embracing Your Journey to Healing

Celebrating Small Victories

Living with Polycystic Ovary Syndrome (PCOS) can feel like an uphill battle at times. The symptoms can be overwhelming and the journey to healing can seem long and daunting. However, it's important to remember to celebrate the small victories along the way. These victories can be a reminder of how far you've come and can provide motivation to keep pushing forward on your journey to healing.

One small victory to celebrate could be sticking to a healthy diet for a week. Making dietary changes can be challenging, especially when cravings for sugary and processed foods are strong. By sticking to a diet rich in whole foods, you are nourishing your body and supporting your hormones, which is a huge step towards healing PCOS naturally.

Another small victory to celebrate could be incorporating regular exercise into your routine. Exercise has been shown to help regulate hormones and improve insulin sensitivity, both of which are crucial for managing PCOS symptoms. Whether it's going for a walk, practicing yoga, or hitting the gym, finding a form of exercise that you enjoy and can stick to is a victory worth celebrating.

Additionally, celebrating small victories can help shift your mindset from focusing on what you haven't achieved yet to recognizing and acknowledging the progress you've made. This positive mindset can help boost your confidence and motivation to continue making positive changes in your life. Remember, healing PCOS naturally is a journey, not a destination, and every small victory is a step in the right direction.

In conclusion, celebrating small victories is a crucial part of the healing process for people with PCOS. Whether it's sticking to a healthy diet, incorporating regular exercise, or simply shifting your mindset to one of gratitude and positivity, every small victory is worth celebrating.

By acknowledging and celebrating these victories, you can stay motivated and inspired on your journey to healing PCOS naturally. Remember, you are strong, resilient, and capable of overcoming any obstacle that comes your way.

Finding Joy in the Process

Living with PCOS can be challenging, but it is important to remember that healing is a journey, not a destination. Finding joy in the process of healing can make a world of difference in your overall well-being. Instead of focusing solely on the end goal of managing your symptoms, try to find happiness in the small victories along the way.

One way to find joy in the process of healing PCOS naturally is to celebrate the progress you make, no matter how small it may seem. Whether it's incorporating more whole foods into your diet, finding an exercise routine that works for you, or simply taking time for self-care, every step you take towards better health is a reason to rejoice.

Another way to find joy in the process is to surround yourself with a supportive community of people who understand what you're going through. Connecting with others who have PCOS can provide a sense of camaraderie and encouragement, helping you feel less alone in your journey towards healing.

It's also important to practice gratitude for the ways in which your body is already supporting you. Instead of dwelling on the symptoms of PCOS that may be causing you discomfort, try to focus on the things your body does well. By shifting your perspective towards gratitude, you can cultivate a sense of appreciation for the strength and resilience of your body.

Finally, remember to be kind to yourself throughout the healing process. PCOS can be a complex and multifaceted condition, and there may be setbacks along the way. By practicing self-compassion and treating yourself with gentleness and understanding, you can find joy in the process of healing and empower yourself to take control of your health and well-being.

Staying Positive and Focused on Your Goals

Staying positive and focused on your goals is crucial when it comes to managing and healing PCOS naturally. It can be easy to feel overwhelmed and discouraged by the symptoms and challenges that come with this condition, but maintaining a positive mindset is key to staying motivated on your healing journey.

By setting specific goals for yourself and focusing on the steps you need to take to achieve them, you can stay on track and make progress towards better health.

One way to stay positive and focused on your goals is to surround yourself with a supportive community of people who understand what you're going through. This could be friends, family members, or even online support groups for women with PCOS. Having a network of people who can offer encouragement, advice, and motivation can make a huge difference in your ability to stay positive and focused on your healing journey.

In addition to finding support from others, it's important to practice self-care and prioritize your mental and emotional well-being. This could include activities like meditation, journaling, spending time in nature, or engaging in hobbies that bring you joy. Taking care of yourself in this way can help you stay grounded, reduce stress, and maintain a positive outlook as you work towards healing your PCOS naturally.

Another important aspect of staying positive and focused on your goals is to celebrate your successes, no matter how small they may seem. Whether you've made progress in changing your diet, incorporating more exercise into your routine, or reducing stress in your life, it's important to acknowledge and celebrate these achievements. Recognizing your progress can help you stay motivated and inspired to continue making positive changes in your life.

Finally, remember that healing PCOS naturally is a journey, and it's important to be patient and kind to yourself along the way. There will be ups and downs, setbacks and breakthroughs, but by staying positive, focused, and committed to your goals, you can overcome the challenges of PCOS and create a healthier, happier life for yourself. Stay motivated, stay positive, and never give up on your journey to healing PCOS naturally.

Empowering Yourself to Take Control of Your Health

Empowering yourself to take control of your health is essential when it comes to managing PCOS naturally. By understanding the underlying causes of this condition and making informed choices about your diet, lifestyle, and treatment options, you can significantly improve your symptoms and overall well-being. It's important to remember that you are not alone in this journey, and there are many resources and support networks available to help you along the way.

One of the first steps in empowering yourself to take control of your health is to educate yourself about PCOS and its impact on your body. By learning about the hormonal imbalances, insulin resistance, and other factors that contribute to this condition, you can make more informed decisions about your treatment plan.

This knowledge will also help you advocate for yourself when discussing your health with healthcare providers and seeking out alternative therapies.

Another key aspect of taking control of your health with PCOS is making positive changes to your diet and lifestyle. Eating a balanced diet rich in whole foods, exercising regularly, and managing stress can all have a significant impact on your symptoms and help regulate your hormones.

By taking a proactive approach to your health, you can reduce inflammation, improve insulin sensitivity, and support your body's natural healing processes.

In addition to making changes to your diet and lifestyle, it's important to explore alternative therapies and treatments that can help manage your PCOS symptoms. Acupuncture, herbal medicine, and supplements are just a few examples of natural approaches that have been shown to be effective in supporting hormone balance and alleviating symptoms.

By working with a qualified practitioner who specializes in treating PCOS, you can tailor a treatment plan that is personalized to your unique needs and goals.

Overall, empowering yourself to take control of your health with PCOS is a journey that requires dedication, patience, and self-compassion. By educating yourself, making positive changes to your diet and lifestyle, and exploring alternative therapies, you can improve your symptoms and quality of life. Remember that you are the expert on your own body, and by taking an active role in your health, you can create a path to healing that is sustainable and empowering.

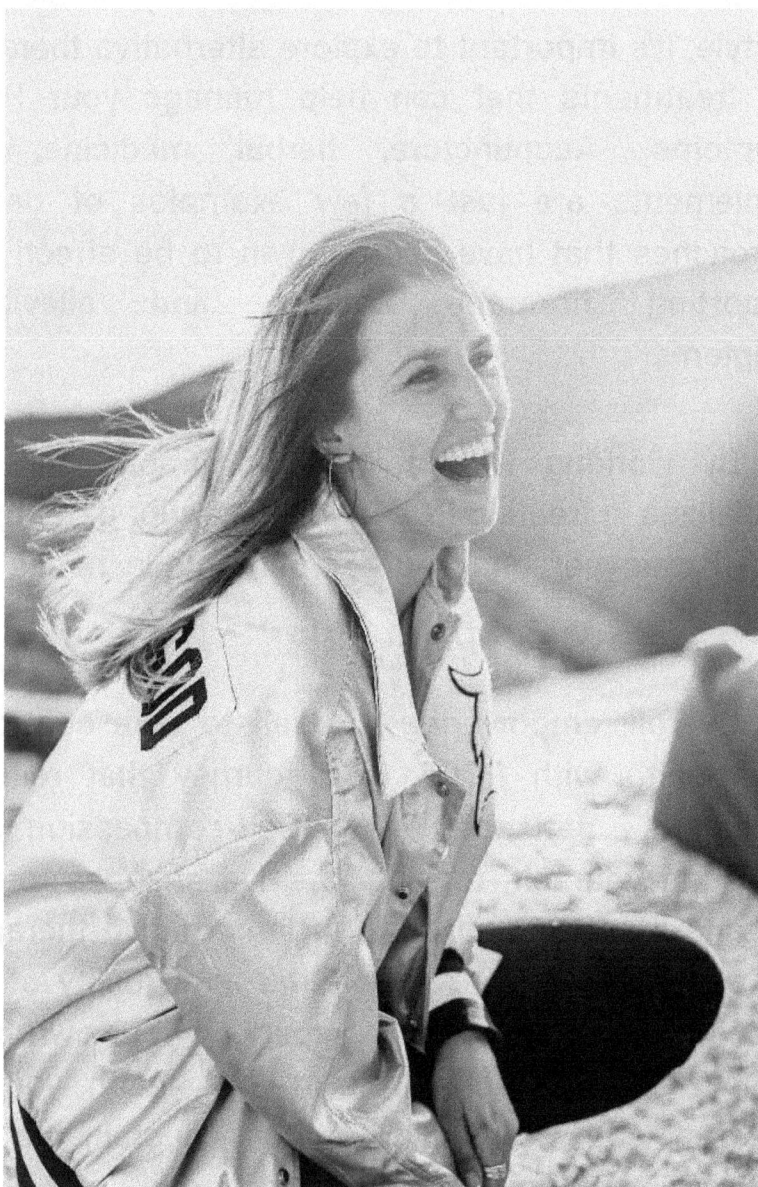

Chapter 10

Resources for Women with PCOS

Books, Websites, and Support Groups

In your journey to heal PCOS naturally, it is essential to educate yourself on the condition. Books are a great resource for gaining in-depth knowledge about PCOS, its symptoms, causes, and natural treatment options.

Some recommended books for women with PCOS include "The PCOS Solution" by Colette Harris and Theresa Cheung, "8 Steps to Reverse Your PCOS" by Fiona McCulloch, and "The Hormone Cure" by Dr. Sara Gottfried. These books provide valuable insights and practical tips on managing PCOS and improving your overall health.

Websites are another valuable resource for women with PCOS looking to educate themselves and connect with others who are facing similar challenges. Some reputable websites that offer information and support for women with PCOS include PCOS Diva, PCOS Nutrition Center, and the National Institute of Diabetes and Digestive and Kidney Diseases (NIDDK) website.

These websites offer a wealth of resources, including articles, recipes, forums, and online support groups where you can connect with other women with PCOS.

Support groups can be a lifeline for women with PCOS, providing emotional support, encouragement, and practical advice on managing the condition. Joining a support group can help you feel less alone in your journey and provide you with a sense of community. Look for local support groups in your area or consider joining online support groups on social media platforms like Facebook. Connecting with other women who understand what you're going through can be empowering and motivating as you work towards healing PCOS naturally.

In addition to books, websites, and support groups, it is important to consult with healthcare professionals who specialize in treating PCOS naturally. A naturopathic doctor, functional medicine practitioner, or holistic healthcare provider can help you create a personalized treatment plan that addresses the root causes of your PCOS and promotes healing from within.

These healthcare professionals can offer guidance on dietary changes, supplements, lifestyle modifications, and natural therapies that can help balance your hormones and alleviate PCOS symptoms.

Remember, healing PCOS naturally is a journey that requires patience, persistence, and self-care. By educating yourself, connecting with others, and seeking support from healthcare professionals, you can take control of your health and well-being. Embrace the power of knowledge, community, and natural healing as you work towards healing PCOS and reclaiming your vitality and vitality.

Finding Healthcare Providers who Understand PCOS

Finding healthcare providers who understand PCOS can be a challenging task for many women. PCOS is a complex and often misunderstood condition, so it is important to seek out healthcare professionals who are knowledgeable and experienced in treating this condition.

When looking for a healthcare provider, it is essential to do your research and find someone who is familiar with the latest research and treatment options for PCOS.

One of the first steps in finding a healthcare provider who understands PCOS is to ask for recommendations from other women who have the condition. Many women with PCOS have found success in working with healthcare providers who have experience in treating this condition. You can also ask your primary care physician for recommendations or search online for healthcare providers in your area who specialize in treating PCOS.

When meeting with a potential healthcare provider, be sure to ask about their experience in treating PCOS and their approach to managing the condition. It is important to find a healthcare provider who takes a holistic approach to treating PCOS and is willing to work with you to develop a personalized treatment plan that addresses your individual needs and concerns.

Look for a healthcare provider who is open to discussing lifestyle changes, dietary modifications, and natural treatment options in addition to traditional medical interventions.

It is also important to find a healthcare provider who listens to your concerns and takes the time to answer your questions. PCOS can have a significant impact on your physical and emotional well-being, so it is important to find a healthcare provider who is compassionate and understanding. A good healthcare provider will work with you to address your symptoms and help you manage your condition in a way that is sustainable and effective.

In conclusion, finding healthcare providers who understand PCOS is essential for women who are looking to manage their condition and improve their overall health and well-being. By doing your research, asking for recommendations, and seeking out healthcare providers who take a holistic approach to treating PCOS, you can find a provider who will work with you to develop a personalized treatment plan that meets your needs.

Remember that you are your own best advocate, so don't be afraid to ask questions and seek out healthcare providers who are willing to listen to your concerns and work with you to find effective solutions for managing your PCOS.

Recommended Products for PCOS Management

If you have PCOS, managing your symptoms can be a challenging task. However, there are various products available that can help you in your journey towards healing PCOS naturally. In this subchapter, we will discuss some recommended products that can aid in managing the symptoms of PCOS and promoting overall wellness.

One essential product for PCOS management is a high-quality multivitamin. Women with PCOS often have nutrient deficiencies, so taking a multivitamin can help ensure that your body is getting the necessary vitamins and minerals it needs to function properly. Look for a multivitamin specifically formulated for women with PCOS, as it may contain additional nutrients that are beneficial for managing the condition.

Another recommended product for PCOS management is a good quality omega-3 supplement. Omega-3 fatty acids have been shown to help reduce inflammation in the body, which can be beneficial for women with PCOS who often experience high levels of inflammation. Omega-3 supplements can also help improve insulin sensitivity and regulate menstrual cycles, making them a valuable addition to your PCOS management routine.

In addition to supplements, incorporating a high-quality probiotic into your daily routine can also be beneficial for managing PCOS symptoms. Probiotics help promote a healthy gut microbiome, which is important for overall health and hormonal balance.

A healthy gut can also improve digestion and nutrient absorption, which can be beneficial for women with PCOS who often experience digestive issues.

For managing PCOS symptoms related to insulin resistance, a good quality chromium supplement can be helpful. Chromium is a mineral that plays a role in insulin sensitivity and glucose metabolism, making it a valuable supplement for women with PCOS who struggle with insulin resistance. Adding a chromium supplement to your daily routine may help improve blood sugar control and reduce symptoms associated with insulin resistance.

Lastly, incorporating adaptogenic herbs such as ashwagandha or rhodiola into your routine can help support your body's stress response and hormone balance. Adaptogens can help reduce stress levels, improve energy levels, and promote overall well-being, making them a valuable addition to your PCOS management routine. By incorporating these recommended products into your daily routine, you can support your body in managing PCOS symptoms naturally and promoting overall health and wellness.

Continuing Your Education and Advocacy for PCOS Awareness

Education is key in managing and treating PCOS naturally. By continuing to educate yourself about the condition, you can stay informed about the latest research, treatments, and lifestyle changes that can help improve your symptoms. There are many resources available, including books, websites, support groups, and healthcare providers who specialize in PCOS. By staying informed, you can make informed decisions about your health and well-being.

Advocacy for PCOS awareness is also important in helping to reduce the stigma surrounding the condition and increase funding for research and treatment options. By sharing your story and raising awareness about PCOS, you can help other women who may be struggling with similar symptoms. You can also advocate for better access to healthcare and support for women with PCOS, both in your community and on a larger scale.

One way to advocate for PCOS awareness is to participate in events and campaigns that raise awareness about the condition. This can include participating in walks, runs, or other fundraisers, or sharing your story on social media or in local newspapers. By speaking out about your experiences with PCOS, you can help to break down barriers and empower other women to seek help and support.

In addition to education and advocacy, it's important to continue taking care of yourself and prioritizing your health. This includes following a healthy diet, getting regular exercise, managing stress, and getting regular check-ups with your healthcare provider. By taking control of your health and making positive lifestyle changes, you can help to manage your symptoms and improve your overall well-being.

Remember, you are not alone in your journey with PCOS. By continuing your education, advocating for awareness, and taking care of yourself, you can empower yourself to live a healthier, happier life with PCOS. Keep pushing forward, seeking support from others, and never give up on your journey to healing PCOS naturally.

Author Notes & Acknowledgments

First and foremost, I would like to express my deepest gratitude to the people who inspired and supported me throughout the journey of writing this book. This project would not have been possible without their unwavering belief in me and their invaluable contributions.

To my wife, thank you for your constant encouragement and understanding. Your love and support have been my anchor during the challenging times of researching and writing this book. Your belief in my ability to make a difference in people's lives has been my driving force.

I would also like to disclose that this book contains some renewed artificial intelligence-generated content. I really appreciate very recent technological innovation by outstanding scientists and of course our reader's understanding.

Lastly, I want to express my deepest gratitude to the readers of this book. I sincerely hope the strategies and methods outlined within these pages will provide you with the knowledge and tools needed to truly make your life much better. Your commitment to seeking any good solutions and willingness to explore multiple methods is commendable.

Author Bio

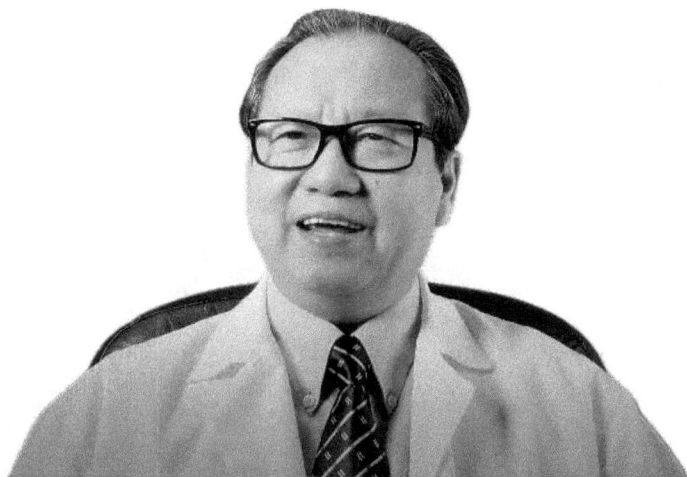

Johnson Wu earned his MD in 1982. With over 40 years of clinical experience, he has worked in hospitals in Zhejiang and Shanghai, China, as well as the Royal Marsden Hospital (part of Imperial College) in London, UK. Upon the recommendation of Sir Aaron Klug, the president of The Royal Society and a Nobel Prize winner in Chemistry, Dr. Wu was honorably awarded a British Royal Society Fellowship. He has published over 100 medical books in many countries and currently practices medicine in Canada.